HEART HEALTHY RECIPES FOR SENIORS
Nutritious Recipes for Active Aging

GEORGE S. MILLS

TABLE OF CONTENT

INTRODUCTION

A heart-healthy diet is an eating plan that focuses on fruits, vegetables, whole grains, high-fiber foods, lean proteins, and healthy fats. This type of diet helps to reduce the risk of heart disease, stroke, and other health conditions. Eating a heart-healthy diet can also reduce the risk of developing type 2 diabetes and improve overall health.

To start a heart-healthy diet, it is important to focus on eating nutrient-rich foods. This means prioritizing foods that are high in vitamins and minerals, like fruits, vegetables, whole grains, lean proteins, and healthy fats. It is also important to limit processed and refined foods that are high in saturated fat, trans fat, sodium, and added sugar.

Fruits and vegetables are an important part of a heart-healthy diet. Fruits and vegetables are packed with vitamins, minerals, fiber, and antioxidants. Aim to fill half of your plate with fruits and vegetables at every meal. Choose a variety of colorful fruits and vegetables to ensure you get a wide range of nutrients.

Whole grains are another important part of a heart-healthy diet. Whole grains are high in fiber and other nutrients, like B vitamins and magnesium. Aim to make at least half of the grains you eat whole grains, like whole wheat bread, oats, quinoa, and brown rice. In addition to fruits, vegetables, and whole grains, it is important to include lean proteins in your diet. Lean proteins, like fish, poultry, beans, and lentils, are low in saturated fat and contain important nutrients like iron and zinc.

Healthy fats are an important part of a heart-healthy diet. Healthy fats, like those found in nuts, seeds, avocados, and olive oil, help keep cholesterol levels in check and provide essential fatty acids. Aim to limit saturated and trans fats, which are found in fried and processed foods.

Finally, it is important to limit processed and refined foods. These foods are often high in sodium, sugar, and unhealthy fats. Try to limit packaged snacks and fast food and choose fresh, whole foods instead.

As you start to make changes to your diet, it is important to keep the guidelines of a heart-healthy diet in mind. Aim to fill half of your plate with fruits and vegetables, make at least half of your grains whole grains, include lean proteins, and limit processed and refined foods. A heart-healthy diet can help reduce your risk of heart disease and other health conditions.

As we age, it can become increasingly difficult to maintain a healthy lifestyle. Many seniors become increasingly sedentary, and their dietary habits can suffer as well. This can lead to an increased risk of heart disease, stroke, and other conditions, which can have a significant impact on their quality of life. Fortunately, there are a variety of heart-healthy recipes that can help seniors eat healthily and stay active.

These heart-healthy recipes are specifically tailored to the needs of seniors, providing them with the nutrition and energy that they need to stay healthy. These recipes are designed to be both nutritious and delicious, making them a great option for those who want to enjoy their meals without compromising their health. Additionally, these recipes are often easy to make and require minimal time and effort, making them an ideal choice for busy seniors.

These recipes are also cost-effective, which is important for many seniors who may be on a limited budget. Furthermore, many of these recipes can be enjoyed as part of a larger meal, making them a great way to add variety to meals without compromising nutrition. Overall, heart-healthy recipes for seniors are an excellent way to ensure that seniors are getting the nutrition they need while still enjoying delicious meals. With these recipes, seniors can enjoy a variety of nutritious meals while reducing their risk of heart disease and other conditions.

BREAKFAST RECIPES

1. Oatmeal with Fresh Berries and Nuts
2. Egg White and Vegetable Omelet
3. High-Fiber Whole-Grain Toast with Avocado and Egg
4. Greek Yogurt Parfait with Fresh Fruit
5. Baked Sweet Potato with Sunflower Seeds
6. Overnight Oats with Apples and Cinnamon
7. Salmon and Spinach Frittata
8. Quinoa Porridge with Almonds and Raisins
9. Smoothie Bowl with Chia Seeds and Berries
10. Egg and Veggie Scramble
11. Kale and Mushroom Egg White Omelet
12. Fruit and Nut Granola
13. Peanut Butter-Banana-Oat Breakfast Wrap
14. Sweet Potato and Egg Hash
15. Vegetable-Egg Frittata Muffins
16. Steel-Cut Oats with Berries and Flaxseed

17. Breakfast Burrito with Black Beans and Egg Whites
18. Avocado Toast with Poached Eggs
19. Zucchini and Cheese Omelet
20. Banana-Almond Butter Toast with Chia Seeds

Oatmeal with Fresh Berries and Nuts

Ingredients:
-1 cup of rolled oats
-1 cup of fresh berries (strawberries, blueberries, raspberries, etc)
-1/4 cup of chopped nuts (almonds, walnuts, pecans, etc)
-1 cup of milk
-1 teaspoon of honey

Meal Preparation:
1. In a medium saucepan, heat the milk over medium-high heat until it begins to simmer.
2. Reduce the heat to low, add the rolled oats, and simmer for 5 minutes, stirring occasionally.
3. Add the honey and stir until it is fully incorporated.
4. Remove the oatmeal from the heat and stir in the fresh berries and chopped nuts.
5. Serve warm with additional honey or milk, if desired.
Prep Time: 10 minutes

Egg White and Vegetable Omelet
Ingredients:
- 2 large egg whites
- 1/4 cup chopped onions
- 1/4 cup chopped bell peppers
- 2 tablespoons chopped mushrooms
- 1/4 teaspoon dried oregano
- 2 teaspoons olive oil
- Salt and pepper to taste

Meal Preparation:
1. Heat olive oil in a skillet over medium heat.

2. Add onions, bell peppers, mushrooms, and oregano. Cook for about 3 minutes, stirring often.
3. Add the egg whites to the skillet. Stir and cook until the egg whites are set.
4. Season with salt and pepper.
5. Serve the omelet with your favorite sides.
Prep Time: 10 minutes

High-Fiber Whole-Grain Toast with Avocado and Egg

Ingredients:
- 2 slices of whole-grain bread
- 1/2 ripe avocado
- 1/4 teaspoon kosher salt
- 2 eggs
- 2 teaspoons extra-virgin olive oil
- 1/4 teaspoon freshly ground black pepper

Meal Preparation:
1. Preheat the oven to 375 degrees Fahrenheit.
2. Toast the whole-grain bread in the oven for 8-10 minutes, or until golden brown and crisp.
3. Meanwhile, mash the avocado in a small bowl and season with the kosher salt.
4. Heat the olive oil in a large non-stick skillet over medium-high heat.
5. Crack the eggs into the skillet and season with the pepper. Cook for 3-4 minutes, or until the eggs are cooked to your desired doneness.
6. To assemble, spread the mashed avocado on the toasted bread and top with the cooked eggs.
Prep Time: 20 minutes
Greek Yogurt Parfait with Fresh Fruit

Ingredients:
-1 cup of Greek yogurt

-1 tablespoon honey
-1/2 cup of fresh blueberries
-1/2 cup of fresh raspberries
-1/4 cup of chopped almonds

Meal Preparation:
1. In a medium bowl, combine the Greek yogurt and honey and mix until combined.
2. In a separate bowl, mix together the blueberries and raspberries.
3. Layer the yogurt mixture and fruit in a parfait glass, alternating between the yogurt and fruit.
4. Top with chopped almonds.
5. Serve and enjoy!
Prep Time: 10 minute

Baked Sweet Potato with Sunflower Seeds

Ingredients:
-1 large sweet potato
-1 tablespoon olive oil
-1/2 teaspoon salt
-1 tablespoon sunflower seeds

Meal Preparation:
1. Preheat the oven to 375°F.
2. Wash and scrub the sweet potato, then place it on a baking sheet.
3. Drizzle the olive oil over the sweet potato and sprinkle with salt.
4. Bake for 45 minutes, or until the sweet potato is tender.
5. Remove from the oven and sprinkle with sunflower seeds. Serve warm.
Prep Time: 10 minutes
Cook Time: 45 minutes

Overnight Oats with Apples and Cinnamon

Ingredients:

-1/2 cup rolled oats
-1/2 cup milk or non-dairy milk
-1/4 cup plain yogurt
-1 small apple, diced
-1 tablespoon honey or maple syrup
-1 teaspoon ground cinnamon
-1/4 teaspoon ground nutmeg
-Pinch of salt

Meal Preparation:
1. In a medium bowl, combine the oats, milk, yogurt, apple, honey, cinnamon, nutmeg, and salt. Stir until everything is evenly distributed.
2. Transfer the mixture to a jar or container and cover with a lid. Refrigerate overnight.
3. In the morning, top the oats with extra diced apples and a sprinkle of cinnamon. Enjoy!
Prep Time: 5 minutes
Chill Time: 8 hours

Salmon and Spinach Frittata

Ingredients:
-2 tablespoons olive oil
-1 pound salmon fillet, skin removed and diced
-1 onion, chopped
-2 cloves garlic, minced
-2 cups fresh spinach, chopped
-6 large eggs
-1/2 cup milk
-1/2 teaspoon salt
-1/4 teaspoon pepper

Meal Preparation:
1. Preheat the oven to 375°F.

2. Heat the olive oil in a large oven-safe skillet over medium-high heat.
3. Add the diced salmon, onion and garlic and cook, stirring occasionally, until the salmon is cooked through and the onion is softened, about 5 minutes.
4. Add the spinach and cook until wilted, about 2 minutes.
5. In a large bowl, whisk together the eggs, milk, salt and pepper.
6. Pour the egg mixture into the skillet and stir to combine.
7. Bake in the preheated oven for 30 minutes, or until the frittata is golden brown and set.
Prep Time: 15 minutes
Cook Time: 30 minutes

Quinoa Porridge with Almonds and Raisins

Ingredients:
-1/2 cup quinoa
-1/4 cup raisins
-1/4 cup slivered almonds
-3 cups water
-1 teaspoon ground cinnamon
-2 tablespoons honey
-1/4 teaspoon sea salt

Meal Preparation:
1. Rinse quinoa in a fine mesh strainer.
2. In a medium saucepan, combine quinoa, raisins, almonds, water, cinnamon, honey, and sea salt.
3. Bring to a boil and reduce heat to a low simmer.
4. Cover and cook for 15 minutes or until quinoa is cooked through and liquid is absorbed.
5. Remove from heat and let sit for 5 minutes.
6. Serve warm, topped with additional nuts and raisins, if desired.
Prep Time: 20 minutes

Smoothie Bowl with Chia Seeds and Berries

Ingredients:
-1/2 cup of frozen berries (blueberries, raspberries, blackberries, etc)
-1/4 cup of chia seeds
-1/2 cup of milk (dairy, almond, or coconut)
-1 frozen banana
-1 teaspoon of honey (optional)

Meal Preparation:
1. In a blender, combine the frozen berries, chia seeds, milk, banana, and honey (if desired).
2. Blend until smooth.
3. Pour into a bowl and top with additional fresh berries and chia seeds.
Prep Time: 10 minutes

Egg and Veggie Scramble

Ingredients:
- 4 large eggs
- 1/4 cup diced onion
- 2 cups fresh spinach
- 1/4 cup diced tomatoes
- 1/4 cup shredded cheese
- 2 tablespoons of olive oil
- Salt and pepper to taste

Meal Preparation:
1. Heat the olive oil in a large skillet over medium heat.
2. Add the diced onion and sauté for 5 minutes.
3. Add the spinach and tomatoes and cook for an additional 5 minutes.
4. Crack the eggs into the skillet and scramble them with the vegetables.
5. Add the shredded cheese and season with salt and pepper.
6. Cook until the eggs are cooked through and the cheese is melted.
Prep Time: 15 minutes

Kale and Mushroom Egg White Omelet

Ingredients:
- 2 cups of kale, chopped
- ½ cup of mushrooms, chopped
- 6 egg whites
- Salt and pepper to taste
- 2 tablespoons of olive oil

Meal Preparation:
1. Heat the olive oil in a non-stick skillet over medium heat.
2. Add the kale and mushrooms to the skillet and sauté until the vegetables are lightly cooked and tender, about 5 minutes.
3. In a separate bowl, whisk together the egg whites until frothy.
4. Pour the egg whites into the skillet with the vegetables and season with salt and pepper.
5. Cook the omelet until the egg whites are set and the edges are golden brown, about 5 minutes.
6. Flip the omelet over and cook until the other side is golden brown, about 3 minutes.
7. Serve the omelet hot with your favorite toppings.
Prep Time: 15 minutes

Fruit and Nut Granola

Ingredients:
-3 cups old-fashioned rolled oats
-1/4 cup packed brown sugar
-1/4 cup honey
-1/4 cup vegetable oil
-1/2 teaspoon ground cinnamon
-1/2 cup chopped nuts (such as almonds, walnuts, or pecans)
-1/2 cup dried fruit (such as raisins, cranberries, or cherries)

Meal Preparation:

1. Preheat the oven to 300°F.
2. In a large bowl, combine oats, brown sugar, honey, vegetable oil, and cinnamon.
3. Spread the oat mixture on a baking sheet.
4. Bake for 15 minutes, stirring once halfway through.
5. Remove from the oven and stir in nuts and dried fruit.
6. Return to the oven and bake for an additional 15 minutes, stirring once halfway through.
7. Remove from the oven and let cool before serving.
Prep Time: 30 minutes

Peanut Butter-Banana-Oat Breakfast Wrap

Ingredients:
-1/2 cup rolled oats
2 tablespoons peanut butter
-1 banana, sliced
-1 teaspoon cinnamon
-1 teaspoon honey
-1/4 cup almond milk

Meal Preparation:
1. In a medium bowl, combine the oats, peanut butter, cinnamon, and honey.
2. Add the almond milk and mix until all ingredients are combined.
3. Heat a small non-stick skillet over medium heat.
4. Place the banana slices in the skillet and cook for about 2 minutes, or until the bananas are lightly caramelized.
5. Spread the oat mixture on top of the banana slices.
6. Cook for about 2 minutes, or until the oats are golden brown.
7. Flip the wrap and cook for another 2 minutes.
8. Remove from the skillet and enjoy!
Prep Time: 10 minutes

Sweet Potato and Egg Hash

Ingredients:
-2 sweet potatoes, cut into cubes
-2 tablespoons olive oil
-1 onion, diced
-2 cloves garlic, minced
-1 teaspoon smoked paprika
-Salt and pepper to taste
-4 eggs

Meal Preparation:
1. Preheat the oven to 350°F.
2. Toss sweet potatoes in olive oil and spread onto a baking sheet.
3. Bake for 25 minutes, or until potatoes are tender.
4. Heat a large skillet over medium heat.
5. Add olive oil, onion, and garlic to the skillet.
6. Cook for 5 minutes, stirring occasionally.
7. Add paprika, salt, and pepper to the skillet.
8. Add the cooked sweet potatoes and stir to combine.
9. Cook for 5 minutes, stirring occasionally.
10. Crack the eggs into the skillet and cook until the whites are set, about 5 minutes.
Prep Time: 35 minutes

Vegetable-Egg Frittata Muffins

Ingredients:
- 5 large eggs
- 1/4 cup milk
- 1/4 teaspoon black pepper
- 1/4 teaspoon salt
- 1/2 cup diced onion
- 1/2 cup diced bell pepper
- 1 cup chopped kale
- 1/2 cup shredded cheese

Meal Preparation:

1. Preheat the oven to 375 degrees F.
2. In a large bowl, whisk together eggs, milk, pepper, and salt.
3. In a medium skillet, sauté onions, bell pepper, and kale for 5 minutes.
4. Add sautéed vegetables to egg mixture and stir to combine.
5. Grease a 12-muffin tin and divide egg mixture evenly among the muffin cups.
6. Sprinkle cheese on top of each muffin cup.
7. Bake for 20 minutes or until muffins are set.
Prep Time: 25 minutes

Steel-Cut Oats with Berries and Flaxseed

Ingredients:
-1 cup steel-cut oats
-1/2 cup fresh or frozen berries
-1 tablespoon flaxseed
-2 cups water
-Honey or brown sugar, to taste

Meal Preparation:
1. Bring the water to a boil in a medium saucepan.
2. Add the steel-cut oats and reduce the heat to a low simmer.
3. Cook the oats for 15 minutes, stirring occasionally.
4. Remove from heat and stir in the berries, flaxseed, and honey or brown sugar, to taste.
Prep Time: 15 minutes

Breakfast Burrito with Black Beans and Egg Whites
I ngredients:
-4 large whole wheat tortillas
-1/2 cup canned black beans, rinsed and drained
-1/4 cup egg whites
-1/4 cup shredded cheese
-1/4 cup diced onions
-1/4 cup diced tomatoes
-1/4 cup diced bell pepper
-Salt and pepper to taste

Meal Preparation:
1. Preheat a large skillet over medium heat.
2. Spread the beans onto the tortillas, followed by the egg whites, cheese, onions, tomatoes, and bell pepper.
3. Sprinkle it with salt and pepper to taste.
4. Fold the tortillas over to enclose the filling.
5. Place the burritos in the skillet and cook until lightly browned and the filling is hot, about 5 minutes per side.
Prep Time: 10 minutes

Avocado Toast with Poached Eggs

Ingredients:
-2 slices of bread
-1 avocado
-2 eggs
-Salt and pepper
-Olive oil
Meal Preparation:
1. Toast the bread slices in a toaster or in a pan over medium heat.
2. Cut the avocado in half lengthwise and remove the pit. Scoop out the flesh of the avocado and mash it with a fork until it forms a paste.
3. Season the mashed avocado with salt and pepper to taste.
4. Spread the mashed avocado on the toasted bread slices.
5. Heat a pan over medium heat and add some olive oil.
6. Crack the eggs into the pan and cook for 2-3 minutes until the whites are set.
7. Place the poached eggs on top of the avocado toast and sprinkle with salt and pepper.
Prep Time: 10 minutes

Zucchini and Cheese Omelet

Ingredients:

- 2 eggs
- 2 tablespoons of milk
- 1/4 cup of shredded cheese
- 1/4 cup of diced zucchini
- 1 tablespoon of olive oil
- Salt and pepper to taste

Meal Preparation:
1. In a medium bowl, whisk together the eggs and milk until well blended.
2. Heat the olive oil in a medium non-stick skillet over medium-high heat.
3. Add the zucchini and cook until tender, about 5 minutes.
4. Add the egg mixture and sprinkle with the cheese.
5. Cook, stirring occasionally, until the eggs are cooked through and the cheese is melted, about 6 to 8 minutes.
6. Season with salt and pepper to taste.
Prep Time: 10 minutes

Banana-Almond Butter Toast with Chia Seeds

Ingredients:
-2 slices of whole wheat or gluten-free bread
-2 tablespoons of almond butter
-1 banana, sliced
-1 tablespoon of chia seeds

Meal Preparation:
1. Toast the bread slices in a toaster or in a skillet over medium heat until golden brown.
2. Spread the almond butter evenly over the slices of toast.
3. Top the slices of toast with the sliced banana.
4. Sprinkle the chia seeds over the banana slices.
Prep Time: 5 minutes

LUNCH RECIPES

1. Quinoa Salad with Spinach and Apples
2. Lentil Soup with Carrots and Kale
3. Baked Eggplant Parmesan
4. Vegetable-Stuffed Peppers
5. Baked Salmon with Citrus Salsa
6. Grilled Chicken Breast with Roasted Vegetables
7. Turkey and White Bean Chili
8. Baked Oatmeal with Berries and Nuts
9. Whole Wheat Pasta with Tomato Sauce
10. Vegetable Stir-Fry with Brown Rice
11. Chickpea and Spinach Stew
12. Baked Sweet Potato Wedges with Rosemary
13. Roasted Vegetable and Bean Burrito
14. Grilled Vegetable Wraps
15. Mediterranean Quinoa Bowl
16. Egg Salad with Avocado and Sprouts
17. Stuffed Acorn Squash with Quinoa and Kale
18. Salmon and Brown Rice Cakes
19. Kale and White Bean Salad
20. Zucchini and Spinach Frittata
21. Bean and Barley Stew
22. Baked Tilapia with Lemon and Herbs
23. Stuffed Peppers with Brown Rice and Lentils
24. Lentil and Tomato Soup
25. Tomato, Avocado and Basil Salad

Quinoa Salad with Spinach and Apples

Ingredients:
-1 cup quinoa
-2 cups spinach
-1 apple, diced

-1/4 cup dried cranberries
-1/4 cup slivered almonds
-1/4 cup olive oil
-1 tablespoon lemon juice
-Salt and pepper to taste

Meal Preparation:
1. Rinse quinoa in a fine mesh strainer.
2. Bring 2 cups of water to a boil in a medium saucepan.
3. Add quinoa to the boiling water and reduce heat to low. Cook for 15 minutes.
4. Remove from heat and fluff with a fork.
5. Place quinoa in a large bowl and add spinach, apple, dried cranberries, and slivered almonds.
6. In a separate bowl, whisk together olive oil, lemon juice, salt, and pepper.
7. Pour dressing over quinoa mixture and mix until combined.
Prep Time: 20 minutes

Lentil Soup with Carrots and Kale

Ingredients:
-1 cup lentils
-1 onion, chopped
-3 cloves garlic, minced
-2 carrots, chopped
-2 cups kale, chopped
-4 cups vegetable broth
-1 teaspoon dried thyme
-1 bay leaf
-Salt and pepper, to taste

Meal Preparation:
1. In a large pot, heat some oil over medium heat.
2. Add the onion and garlic and sauté until softened, about 5 minutes.

3. Add the carrots and sauté for another 3 minutes.
4. Add the lentils, vegetable broth, kale, thyme, and bay leaf.
5. Increase the heat and bring to a boil, then reduce the heat to low, cover, and simmer for 30 minutes.
6. Season with salt and pepper, to taste.
7. Serve hot.

Prep Time: 10 minutes
Cook Time: 30 minutes
Total Time: 40 minutes

Baked Eggplant Parmesan

Ingredients:
2 medium eggplants, sliced into 1/2-inch rounds
1/2 cup olive oil
1 teaspoon salt
1/2 teaspoon freshly ground black pepper
1/4 cup all-purpose flour
2 large eggs, lightly beaten
2 cups Italian-style bread crumbs
2 cups grated Parmesan cheese
1 (24-ounce) jar marinara sauce

Meal Preparation:
1. Preheat the oven to 375 degrees F.
2. Arrange the eggplant slices in a single layer on a baking sheet and brush each slice with the olive oil. Sprinkle with salt and pepper.
3. Place the flour, eggs, and bread crumbs in three separate shallow dishes. Dip each eggplant slice in the flour, then the egg, and then the bread crumbs. Place each coated slice on a baking sheet.
4. Bake for 15 minutes, then turn each slice over and bake for 15 minutes more.
5. In a 9x13-inch baking dish, spread 1/2 cup of the marinara sauce in the bottom of the dish. Arrange the eggplant slices in a single layer on top of the sauce.

6. Top with the remaining sauce and sprinkle with the Parmesan
cheese.
7. Bake for 25 minutes, or until the cheese is melted and bubbly.
Prep Time: 30 minutes

Vegetable-Stuffed Peppers

Ingredients:
-1/2 cup uncooked brown rice
-1 tablespoon olive oil
-1 small onion, chopped
-1 clove garlic, minced
-1 bell pepper, seeded and chopped
-1 cup frozen chopped spinach, thawed and drained
-1 cup canned diced tomatoes
-1 teaspoon Italian seasoning
-1/4 teaspoon salt
-4 large bell peppers, halved and seeded
-1/2 cup shredded mozzarella cheese

Meal Preparation:
1. Preheat the oven to 350 degrees F.
2. In a medium saucepan, cook the rice according to package
directions.
3. Heat the oil in a large skillet over medium heat. Add the onion,
garlic, and bell pepper and cook, stirring often, until the vegetables
are tender, about 5 minutes.
4. Add the spinach, tomatoes, Italian seasoning, and salt to the skillet
and stir to combine. Cook for an additional 5 minutes.
5. Add the cooked rice to the skillet and stir to combine.
6. Place the bell pepper halves in a 9x13 inch baking dish.
7. Fill each bell pepper half with the rice mixture and top with the
mozzarella cheese.
8. Bake for 20 minutes or until the cheese is melted and the peppers
are tender.
Prep Time: 15 minutes
Cook Time: 20 minutes

Total Time: 35 minutes

Baked Salmon with Citrus Salsa

Ingredients:
- 4 salmon fillets
- 2 tablespoons olive oil
- 2 oranges, peeled and diced
- 2 tablespoons red onion, finely chopped
- 2 tablespoons fresh parsley, finely chopped
- Juice of 1/2 lime
- Salt and pepper, to taste

Meal Preparation:
1. Preheat the oven to 400 degrees F.
2. Place the salmon fillets on a baking sheet lined with parchment paper.
3. Drizzle the olive oil over the salmon and season with salt and pepper.
4. Bake for 12-15 minutes, or until the salmon is cooked through.
5. Meanwhile, in a medium bowl, combine the oranges, red onion, parsley, lime juice, and a pinch of salt and pepper.
6. Once the salmon is cooked, top with the citrus salsa and serve.
Prep Time: 15 minutes

Grilled Chicken Breast with Roasted Vegetables

Ingredients:
-4 boneless, skinless chicken breasts
-1 teaspoon garlic powder
-1 teaspoon onion powder
-1 teaspoon paprika
-1/2 teaspoon salt
-1/2 teaspoon black pepper
-2 tablespoons olive oil
-1 red bell pepper, sliced

-1 green bell pepper, sliced
-1 yellow onion, sliced
-1 zucchini, sliced
-1/4 teaspoon Italian seasoning

Meal Preparation:
1. Preheat oven to 425°F.
2. In a small bowl, mix together garlic powder, onion powder, paprika, salt and pepper.
3. Rub the mixture into the chicken breasts.
4. Heat olive oil in a large skillet over medium-high heat.
5. Add chicken breasts and cook until golden brown and cooked through, about 5 minutes per side.
6. Transfer chicken to a baking sheet.
7. In the same skillet, add bell peppers, onion, zucchini, and Italian seasoning.
8. Sauté until vegetables are tender, about 5 minutes.
9. Transfer vegetables to the baking sheet with the chicken.
10. Place the baking sheet in the preheated oven and roast for 15 minutes.
Prep Time: 15 minutes

Turkey and White Bean Chili

Ingredients:

-1 tablespoon olive oil
-1 onion, finely chopped
-2 cloves garlic, minced
-1 lb ground turkey
-1 tablespoon chili powder
-1 teaspoon ground cumin
-1/2 teaspoon dried oregano
-1/2 teaspoon smoked paprika
-1/4 teaspoon ground cinnamon
-1/4 teaspoon cayenne pepper

-1 (15-ounce) can white beans, drained and rinsed
-1 (14.5-ounce) can diced tomatoes
-1 (14.5-ounce) can tomato sauce
-1/2 cup water
-Salt and freshly ground black pepper, to taste
-Chopped fresh parsley, for garnish

Meal Preparation:
1. Heat oil in a large pot over medium heat. Add onion and garlic and cook, stirring occasionally, until softened, about 5 minutes.
2. Add ground turkey and cook, breaking up the meat with a wooden spoon, until browned, about 5 minutes.
3. Add chili powder, cumin, oregano, smoked paprika, cinnamon and cayenne pepper and cook, stirring, for 1 minute.
4. Add white beans, diced tomatoes, tomato sauce and water and stir to combine. Bring to a boil, reduce heat and simmer, stirring occasionally, until slightly thickened, about 20 minutes.
5. Season with salt and pepper, to taste.
6. Serve chili garnished with parsley.
Prep Time: 25 minutes

Baked Oatmeal with Berries and Nuts

Ingredients:
- 2 cups rolled oats
- 1 teaspoon baking powder
- 1/2 teaspoon salt
- 2 tablespoons maple syrup
- 2 tablespoons melted coconut oil
- 2 teaspoons vanilla extract
- 1/2 teaspoon cinnamon
- 1/2 cup chopped almonds
- 1/2 cup chopped walnuts
- 2 cups mixed berries

Meal Preparation:
1. Preheat oven to 350°F (177°C).

2. In a large bowl, combine oats, baking powder, salt, cinnamon, almonds, and walnuts.
3. In a small bowl, whisk together maple syrup, coconut oil, and vanilla extract.
4. Pour the wet ingredients over the dry ingredients and mix together until everything is well combined.
5. Grease an 8x8 inch baking dish with coconut oil and spread the oat mixture into the pan.
6. Top with mixed berries.
7. Bake for 25 minutes or until the oats are golden brown and the berries are bubbling.
Prep Time: 10 minutes
Cook Time: 25 minutes

Whole Wheat Pasta with Tomato Sauce

Ingredients:
- 1/2 lb whole wheat pasta
- 1 28-ounce can diced tomatoes
- 2 cloves garlic, minced
- 1/4 cup extra-virgin olive oil
- 1 teaspoon dried oregano
- Salt and freshly ground black pepper, to taste

Meal Preparation:
1. Bring a large pot of salted water to a boil. Add the pasta and cook until al dente, about 8 minutes. Drain and set aside.
2. In a large skillet, heat the olive oil over medium heat. Add the garlic and cook until fragrant, about 1 minute.
3. Add the tomatoes, oregano, salt, and pepper. Bring to a simmer and cook until the sauce is thickened, about 5 minutes.
4. Add the cooked pasta to the sauce and stir to combine. Serve.
Prep Time: 15 minutes

Vegetable Stir-Fry with Brown Rice

Ingredients:

- 2 tablespoons olive oil
- 1/2 yellow onion, diced
- 1 red bell pepper, diced
- 1 cup mushrooms, sliced
- 1/2 cup frozen peas
- 1/2 cup frozen corn
- 2 cloves garlic, minced
- 2 tablespoons soy sauce
- 1 teaspoon sesame oil
- 1 tablespoon honey
- 2 cups cooked brown rice

Meal Preparation:
1. Heat olive oil in a large skillet over medium heat.
2. Add diced onion, bell pepper, and mushrooms. Cook until vegetables are tender, about 5 minutes.
3. Add frozen peas and corn. Cook for another 3-4 minutes.
4. Add garlic, soy sauce, sesame oil, and honey. Stir to combine.
5. Add cooked brown rice to the skillet and stir to combine.
6. Serve warm.
Prep Time: 15 minutes

Chickpea and Spinach Stew

Ingredients:
-1 onion, chopped
-2 cloves garlic, minced
-1 can (15 ounces) chickpeas, drained and rinsed
-1 can (14.5 ounces) diced tomatoes
-2 cups vegetable broth
-1 teaspoon ground cumin
-1 teaspoon ground coriander
-1/2 teaspoon ground turmeric
-1/4 teaspoon ground cinnamon
-1/4 teaspoon ground black pepper
-2 cups baby spinach

Meal Preparation:
1. In a large saucepan over medium heat, heat oil.
2. Add onion and garlic and cook until softened, about 5 minutes.
3. Add chickpeas, diced tomatoes, vegetable broth, cumin, coriander, turmeric, cinnamon, and black pepper. Bring to a boil, then reduce heat and simmer for 15 minutes.
4. Add spinach and cook until wilted, about 2 minutes.
5. Serve warm.
Prep Time: 20 minutes

Baked Sweet Potato Wedges with Rosemary
Ingredients:
- 2 Sweet Potatoes
- 2 tablespoons Olive Oil
- 1 teaspoon Dried Rosemary
- Salt & Pepper

Meal Preparation:
1. Preheat oven to 400°F.
2. Cut each sweet potato into 8 wedges.
3. In a large bowl, combine sweet potatoes, olive oil, rosemary, salt, and pepper.
4. Spread wedges on a baking sheet lined with parchment paper.
5. Bake for 25 minutes, flipping once halfway through.
Prep Time: 10 minutes

Roasted Vegetable and Bean Burrito

Ingredients:
•1 teaspoon olive oil
•1 large red bell pepper, diced
•1 large yellow onion, diced
•2 cloves garlic, minced
•1/2 teaspoon chili powder

•1/2 teaspoon ground cumin
•1/2 teaspoon smoked paprika
•Salt and pepper, to taste
•1 can (15 ounces) black beans, drained and rinsed
•1 cup cooked brown rice
•1/2 cup frozen corn
•4 burrito-size flour tortillas
•1/2 cup grated cheese

Meal Preparation:
1. Preheat oven to 400 degrees F.
2. Heat a large skillet over medium-high heat and add olive oil.
3. Add bell pepper, onion, garlic, chili powder, cumin, smoked paprika, and a pinch of salt and pepper. Cook, stirring occasionally, until vegetables are softened and beginning to brown, about 5 minutes.
4. Add black beans, cooked rice, and frozen corn to the skillet, and stir to combine. Cook for an additional 2 minutes.
5. Lay the tortillas onto a baking sheet and divide the vegetable and bean mixture among them. Sprinkle with cheese.
6. Bake in preheated oven for 12-15 minutes or until the tortillas are lightly browned and the cheese is melted.
Prep Time: 15 minutes

Grilled Vegetable Wraps

Ingredients:
-1 red pepper
-1 yellow pepper
-1 aubergine
-1 red onion
-1 teaspoon olive oil
-Wraps
-Hummus
-Salad leaves

Meal Preparation:

1. Preheat the grill to a medium heat.
2. Cut the peppers, aubergine and onion into thin slices and place on a baking tray.
3. Drizzle the vegetables with the olive oil and mix to coat.
4. Grill the vegetables for 10-15 minutes or until they are softened and lightly browned.
5. Remove from the grill and allow to cool slightly.
6. Spread the wraps with a layer of hummus and top with the grilled vegetables and salad leaves.
7. Roll up the wraps and serve.
Prep Time: 15 minutes

Mediterranean Quinoa Bowl
Ingredients:
- 1/2 cup quinoa
- 2 tablespoons olive oil
- 1/2 cup diced onion
- 1 red bell pepper, diced
- 1/4 teaspoon salt
- 2 cloves garlic, minced
- 1/2 teaspoon dried oregano
- 1/2 teaspoon dried thyme
- 1/4 teaspoon ground black pepper
- 1/4 cup sundried tomatoes, chopped
- 1/4 cup chopped olives
- 1/4 cup crumbled feta cheese

Meal Preparation:
1. Rinse the quinoa in a fine-mesh strainer, then cook according to package instructions.
2. Heat the olive oil in a large skillet over medium heat. Add the onion and bell pepper, and season with salt. Cook, stirring frequently, until the vegetables are softened, about 5 minutes.
3. Add the garlic, oregano, thyme and black pepper, and cook for 1 minute.
4. Add the sundried tomatoes and olives, and cook for 1 minute.

5. Add the cooked quinoa and feta cheese, and stir to combine.
6. Serve warm or cold.
Prep time: 15 minutes

Egg Salad with Avocado and Sprouts

Ingredients:
- 4 eggs
- 1 avocado, diced
- 2 tablespoons mayonnaise
- 1 tablespoon Dijon mustard
- 2 tablespoons chopped fresh dill
- 2 tablespoons chopped fresh chives
- 2 tablespoons diced red onion
- 1/2 cup sprouts
- Salt and pepper to taste

Meal Preparation:
1. Hard-boil the eggs: Place the eggs in a pot and cover with cold water. Bring the water to a boil, then reduce the heat and simmer for 8-10 minutes. Remove the eggs from the pot and place into an ice bath to cool. Peel the eggs and then dice them.
2. In a large bowl, mash the avocado with a fork until it reaches desired consistency.
3. Add the diced eggs, mayonnaise, mustard, dill, chives, red onion, and sprouts to the bowl with the avocado and mix until all ingredients are combined.
4. Season with salt and pepper to taste and serve.
Prep Time: 15 minutes

Stuffed Acorn Squash with Quinoa and Kale

Ingredients:
- 2 acorn squash
- 1 cup quinoa, cooked
- 2 cups kale, chopped

- 2 tablespoons olive oil
- 1/2 teaspoon sea salt
- 1/2 teaspoon pepper
- 1/2 teaspoon garlic powder

Meal Preparation:
1. Preheat oven to 375°F.
2. Cut the acorn squash in half, lengthwise, and scoop out the seeds.
3. Place the squash on a baking sheet and brush the cut side with olive oil.
4. Bake for 30 minutes.
5. Meanwhile, in a large bowl, combine the cooked quinoa, kale, olive oil, sea salt, pepper, and garlic powder.
6. Once the squash is done baking, fill each half with the quinoa and kale mixture.
7. Bake for an additional 10 minutes.
Prep Time: 40 minutes

Salmon and Brown Rice Cakes

Ingredients:
-1 can (14.75 oz) salmon
-1 cup cooked brown rice
-1/4 cup chopped onion
-1/4 cup chopped red pepper
-2 tablespoons chopped fresh parsley
-2 tablespoons mayonnaise
-1/4 teaspoon garlic powder
-1/4 teaspoon ground black pepper
-1 teaspoon olive oil

Meal Preparation:
1. In a medium bowl, combine the salmon, cooked brown rice, onion, red pepper, parsley, mayonnaise, garlic powder and black pepper.
2. Mix until ingredients are well blended.
3. Form salmon and rice mixture into small patties.
4. Heat olive oil in a large skillet over medium heat.

5. Place patties in the skillet and cook for 4-5 minutes on each side, or until golden brown.
Prep Time: 15 minutes

Kale and White Bean Salad

Ingredients:
-1 bunch kale, stemmed and finely chopped
-1 can white beans, drained and rinsed
-1/4 cup red onion, diced
-1/4 cup walnuts, chopped
-3 tablespoons olive oil
-1 tablespoon lemon juice
-1 tablespoon apple cider vinegar
-1 teaspoon honey
-Salt and pepper, to taste

Meal Preparation:
1. In a large bowl, combine the kale, white beans, red onion, and walnuts.
2. In a small bowl, whisk together the olive oil, lemon juice, apple cider vinegar, and honey.
3. Pour the dressing over the kale mixture and toss to combine.
4. Season with salt and pepper, to taste.
Prep Time: 10 minutes

Zucchini and Spinach Frittata

Ingredients:
-2 tablespoons olive oil
-1 small onion, diced
-2 cloves garlic, minced
-2 cups zucchini, diced
-2 cups baby spinach
-6 eggs
-1/4 cup milk
-1/2 teaspoon salt

-1/4 teaspoon pepper
-1/2 cup grated cheese

Meal Preparation:
1. Preheat oven to 375 degrees.
2. In a large skillet, heat oil over medium heat. Add onion and garlic and cook until onion is soft and translucent.
3. Add zucchini and spinach and cook until tender, about 3 minutes.
4. In a medium bowl, whisk together eggs, milk, salt, and pepper.
5. Add egg mixture to skillet, stirring to combine.
6. Pour mixture into a greased 9-inch pie plate or baking dish.
7. Sprinkle cheese over top.
8. Bake for 20-25 minutes, or until the top is golden and the center is set.
Prep Time: 15 minutes

Bean and Barley Stew

Ingredients:
-1 tablespoon olive oil
-1 onion, chopped
-2 carrots, chopped
-2 celery stalks, chopped
-3 cloves garlic, minced
-1 teaspoon dried oregano
-1/2 teaspoon ground cumin
-1/4 teaspoon black pepper
-1/2 teaspoon salt
-1 (14.5 ounce) can diced tomatoes
-4 cups vegetable broth
-3/4 cup quick-cooking barley
-1 (15 ounce) can kidney beans, drained and rinsed

Meal Preparation:
1. Heat olive oil in a large pot over medium heat.
2. Add onion, carrots, celery, and garlic; cook and stir until vegetables are lightly browned, about 8 minutes.

3. Mix in oregano, cumin, pepper, and salt; cook and stir for 1 minute.
4. Pour in diced tomatoes and vegetable broth, stirring to combine. Bring to a boil.
5. Stir in barley and reduce heat to low; cover and simmer until barley is tender, about 15 minutes.
6. Stir in kidney beans; cook and stir until heated through, about 5 minutes.
Prep Time: 25 minutes

Baked Tilapia with Lemon and Herbs

Ingredients:
-2 tilapia fillets
-1/4 teaspoon garlic powder
-1/4 teaspoon dried oregano
-1/4 teaspoon dried basil
-1/4 teaspoon dried thyme
-1 tablespoon olive oil
-1 tablespoon freshly squeezed lemon juice
-Salt and pepper to taste

Meal Preparation:
1. Preheat the oven to 375°F.
2. Place the tilapia fillets on a baking sheet.
3. In a small bowl, mix together the garlic powder, oregano, basil, thyme, olive oil, and lemon juice.
4. Spread the mixture evenly over the top of the tilapia fillets.
5. Bake in the preheated oven for 10-15 minutes, or until the fish is cooked through and flakes easily with a fork.
6. Serve with your favorite sides.
Prep Time: 15 minutes

Stuffed Peppers with Brown Rice and Lentils

Ingredients:

-4 bell peppers
-1 cup cooked brown rice
-1 cup cooked lentils
-1/2 cup diced onion
-1/2 cup diced celery
-1/2 cup diced carrots
-1/2 teaspoon garlic powder
-1 teaspoon dried oregano
-1 teaspoon dried basil
-1 teaspoon smoked paprika
-1/4 teaspoon salt
-1/4 teaspoon black pepper
-1/2 cup vegetable broth

Meal Preparation:
1. Preheat oven to 375 degrees F (190 degrees C).
2. Cut the bell peppers in half lengthwise and remove the seeds and membranes.
3. In a large bowl, combine the cooked brown rice, cooked lentils, diced onion, diced celery, diced carrots, garlic powder, oregano, basil, smoked paprika, salt, and black pepper. Mix until everything is evenly combined.
4. Stuff the mixture into the bell pepper halves and place them in a baking dish.
5. Pour the vegetable broth into the bottom of the baking dish and cover the dish with aluminum foil.
6. Bake for 30 to 40 minutes, until the bell peppers are tender.1
Prep Time: 15 minutes
Cook Time: 30-40 minutes

Lentil and Tomato Soup
Ingredients:
- 1 cup dried lentils
- 2 tablespoons olive oil
- 1 small onion, finely chopped
- 2 cloves garlic, minced

- 2 carrots, diced
- 1 celery stalk, diced
- 1 tablespoon tomato paste
- 5 cups vegetable broth
- 1 (14.5 ounce) can diced tomatoes
- 1 teaspoon dried oregano
- 1/2 teaspoon dried thyme
- Salt and pepper to taste

Meal Preparation:
1. Heat olive oil in a large pot over medium-high heat.
2. Add the onion, garlic, carrots, and celery. Cook until vegetables are softened, about 5 minutes.
3. Add the tomato paste and cook for 1 minute.
4. Add the lentils, vegetable broth, diced tomatoes, oregano, and thyme.
5. Bring to a boil, then reduce heat and simmer for 25 minutes.
6. Puree the soup with an immersion blender or in a blender or food processor until desired consistency is reached.
7. Season with salt and pepper to taste.
Prep time: 10 minutes
Cook time: 25 minutes

Tomato, Avocado and Basil Salad

Ingredients:
- 2 tomatoes (sliced)
- 1 avocado (cubed)
- 1 handful of fresh basil (chopped)
- 2 tablespoons olive oil
- 1 tablespoon balsamic vinegar
- Salt & pepper (to taste)

Meal Preparation:
1. Slice the tomatoes and cube the avocado.
2. Chop the fresh basil.

3. In a small bowl, whisk together the olive oil and balsamic vinegar.
4. In a larger bowl, combine the tomatoes, avocado, and basil.
5. Drizzle the oil and vinegar mixture over the salad.
6. Season with salt and pepper to taste.
Prep Time: 10 minutes

DINNER RECIPES

1. Baked Salmon with Asparagus
2. Zucchini and Mushroom Frittata
3. Spinach and Mushroom Quiche
4. Pumpkin, Lentil and Spinach Stew
5. Grilled Chicken with Avocado Salsa
6. Broiled Tilapia with Tomatoes and Feta Cheese
7. Bean and Vegetable Burrito
8. Teriyaki Tofu and Vegetable Stir Fry
9. Roasted Broccoli and Quinoa Salad
10. Shrimp and Brown Rice Paella
11. Turkey and White Bean Chili
12. Baked Sweet Potato Fries
13. Grilled Vegetable and Farro Salad
14. Turkey and Brown Rice Stuffed Peppers
15. Roasted Cauliflower and Chickpea Curry
16. Grilled Salmon with Kale and Lemon
17. Stuffed Acorn Squash
18. Lentil and Spinach Soup
19. Quinoa and Black Bean Burger
20. Baked Apples with Walnuts and Cinnamon
21. Wild Rice and Mushroom Pilaf
22. Butternut Squash Risotto
23. Roasted Eggplant and Tomato Stacks
24. Turkey and Vegetable Meatloaf

Baked Salmon with Asparagus

Ingredients:
•1 lb. salmon fillet
•1 bunch asparagus
•2 tablespoons olive oil
•1 teaspoon garlic powder
•1 teaspoon dried parsley
•Salt and pepper

Meal Preparation:
1. Preheat oven to 425°F.
2. Line a baking sheet with parchment paper.
3. Place the salmon fillet on the parchment paper.
4. Drizzle the olive oil over the salmon.
5. Sprinkle garlic powder, parsley, salt, and pepper over the salmon.
6. Place the asparagus around the salmon.
7. Bake for 15-20 minutes, or until the salmon is cooked through.
Prep Time: 10 minutes
Cook Time: 15-20 minutes

Zucchini and Mushroom Frittata

Ingredients:
- 2 tablespoons olive oil
- 1 cup diced zucchini
- 1 cup sliced mushrooms
- 6 large eggs
- 1/4 cup half-and-half
- 1/2 teaspoon freshly ground black pepper
- 1/2 teaspoon dried oregano
- 1/2 teaspoon salt
- 1/2 cup grated Parmesan cheese

Meal Preparation:
1. Preheat oven to 350 degrees F.
2. Heat the olive oil in a large oven-safe skillet over medium heat. Add the zucchini and mushrooms and cook for 5 minutes, stirring occasionally.
3. In a medium bowl, whisk together the eggs, half-and-half, pepper, oregano, and salt.
4. Pour the egg mixture over the vegetables in the skillet and stir to combine.
5. Sprinkle the Parmesan cheese over the top and cook for 5 minutes, stirring occasionally.
6. Place the skillet in the preheated oven and bake for 15 minutes, or until the top is golden brown and the center is set.
7. Let cool for a few minutes before serving.
Prep Time: 25 minutes

Spinach and Mushroom Quiche

Ingredients:
- 2 tablespoons olive oil
- 3 cloves garlic, minced
- 1/2 sweet onion, chopped
- 1 cup mushrooms, sliced
- 2 cups spinach, chopped
- 8 eggs
- 1/4 cup milk
- 1/2 teaspoon salt
- 1/4 teaspoon black pepper
- 1/2 teaspoon thyme
- 1/4 teaspoon nutmeg
- 1 9-inch deep-dish unbaked pastry shell

Meal Preparation:
1. Preheat oven to 350°F.
2. Heat olive oil in a large skillet over medium heat.
3. Add garlic and onion and sauté until onion is softened, about 5 minutes.
4. Add mushrooms and cook until softened, about 5 minutes.

5. Add spinach and cook until wilted, about 2 minutes.
6. In a large bowl, whisk together eggs, milk, salt, pepper, thyme, and nutmeg.
7. Stir in the mushroom-spinach mixture.
8. Pour the egg mixture into the pastry shell.
9. Bake for 40 minutes, or until quiche is set and lightly browned.
Prep Time: 20 minutes
Cook Time: 40 minutes

Pumpkin, Lentil and Spinach Stew

Ingredients:

- 1 tablespoon olive oil
- 1 onion, chopped
- 1 garlic clove, minced
- 1 teaspoon ground cumin
- 1 teaspoon ground coriander
- 1 teaspoon ground ginger
- 1 teaspoon ground turmeric
- 1/2 teaspoon ground cinnamon
- 1/4 teaspoon ground cardamom
- 1/4 teaspoon ground black pepper
- 3 cups vegetable broth
- 1 cup red lentils
- 1 can (15 ounces) pumpkin puree
- 2 cups spinach, chopped

Meal Preparation:
1. Heat the olive oil in a large pot over medium-high heat. Add the onion and cook until softened, about 5 minutes. Add the garlic, cumin, coriander, ginger, turmeric, cinnamon, cardamom, and black pepper and cook until fragrant, about 1 minute.
2. Add the vegetable broth, lentils, and pumpkin puree to the pot. Increase the heat to high and bring the mixture to a boil. Reduce the

heat to low, cover, and simmer until the lentils are tender, about 20 minutes.
3. Add the spinach and cook until wilted, about 5 minutes.
Prep Time:30 minutes

Grilled Chicken with Avocado Salsa

Ingredients:
-2 boneless, skinless chicken breasts
-1 tablespoon olive oil
-salt and pepper, to taste
-1 avocado, diced
-1/4 cup diced red onion
-1/4 cup diced tomato
-1 tablespoon chopped cilantro
-juice of 1/2 lime
-1/4 teaspoon cumin

Meal Preparation:
1. Preheat the grill to medium-high heat.
2. Rub the chicken breasts with the olive oil and season with salt and pepper.
3. Place the chicken on the preheated grill and cook for 4-5 minutes per side, or until cooked through.
4. While the chicken is grilling, prepare the salsa by combining the avocado, red onion, tomato, cilantro, lime juice and cumin in a bowl.
5. Serve the grilled chicken with the avocado salsa.
Prep Time: 10 minutes

Broiled Tilapia with Tomatoes and Feta Cheese

Ingredients:
- 2 tilapia fillets
- 2 tablespoons olive oil
- Salt and pepper, to taste
- 4 Roma tomatoes, diced

- 1/4 cup crumbled feta cheese
- 2 tablespoons fresh chopped parsley

Meal Preparation:
1. Preheat the oven to broil.
2. Place the tilapia fillets on a baking sheet. Drizzle with the olive oil and season with salt and pepper.
3. Broil in the oven for 8-10 minutes or until the fish is cooked through and flaky.
4. Meanwhile, in a small bowl, mix together the diced tomatoes, feta cheese, and parsley.
5. When the fish is cooked, top with the tomato and feta mixture.
6. Broil for an additional 2-3 minutes or until the cheese is melted and bubbly.
7. Serve hot.
Prep Time: 10 minutes
Cook Time: 10 minutes

Bean and Vegetable Burrito

Ingredients:
-1 can (15 ounces) of black beans
-1 can (4 ounces) of diced green chilies
-1 cup frozen corn
-1/2 teaspoon of garlic powder
-2 teaspoons of chili powder
-1/2 teaspoon of cumin
-1/4 teaspoon of salt
-1/4 cup of chopped fresh cilantro
-8 large flour tortillas
-1/2 cup of shredded cheese
-1/2 cup of salsa

Meal Preparation:
1. Drain and rinse the black beans.

2. In a medium saucepan, heat the beans, diced green chilies, frozen corn, garlic powder, chili powder, cumin, and salt. Cook for 5 minutes, stirring occasionally.
3. Remove from heat and stir in the chopped cilantro.
4. Preheat a large skillet over medium heat.
5. Place a tortilla in the skillet and heat until lightly browned and slightly crisp.
6. Flip the tortilla over and spoon a quarter of the bean and vegetable mixture onto one half of the tortilla.
7. Sprinkle with cheese and salsa.
8. Fold the other half of the tortilla over the filling, pressing lightly to seal.
9. Cook until lightly browned, flipping once.
10. Remove from heat and repeat with remaining tortillas.
Prep Time:30 minutes

Teriyaki Tofu and Vegetable Stir Fry

Ingredients:
• 1 package extra-firm tofu, drained and cubed
• 2 tablespoons vegetable oil
• 1 onion, chopped
• 2 cloves garlic, minced
• 1 red bell pepper, seeded and chopped
• 1 head broccoli, cut into florets
• 2 carrots, thinly sliced
• 1/4 cup teriyaki sauce
• 1 tablespoon rice wine vinegar
• 2 tablespoons sesame oil
• 1 tablespoon sesame seeds
• Salt and pepper, to taste

Meal Preparation:
1. Heat vegetable oil in a large skillet over medium-high heat.
2. Add the tofu cubes and cook until golden brown and lightly crisp, about 5 minutes.

3. Add the onion, garlic, bell pepper, broccoli, and carrots to the pan and cook for an additional 5 minutes, stirring occasionally.
4. Add the teriyaki sauce, rice wine vinegar, and sesame oil to the pan and stir to combine.
5. Reduce the heat to medium and simmer for 8-10 minutes, stirring occasionally.
6. Sprinkle with sesame seeds and season with salt and pepper, to taste.
7. Serve over hot cooked rice or noodles.
Prep Time: 15 minutes

Roasted Broccoli and Quinoa Salad

Ingredients:
- 2 cups of quinoa
- 2 heads of broccoli, cut into florets
- 2 tablespoons of olive oil
- 1/4 teaspoon of smoked paprika
- 1/4 teaspoon of garlic powder
- Salt and pepper to taste
- 1/4 cup of toasted pine nuts
- 1/4 cup of crumbled feta cheese
- 1/4 cup of dried cranberries
- 2 tablespoons of freshly chopped parsley
- Juice of 1/2 a lemon

Meal Preparation:
1. Preheat oven to 400 degrees F.
2. In a large bowl, combine quinoa, broccoli florets, olive oil, smoked paprika, garlic powder, salt, and pepper. Mix until everything is evenly coated.
3. Spread the mixture onto a baking sheet and bake for 20 minutes, stirring the mixture once halfway through.
4. Once the quinoa and broccoli are done, transfer to a large bowl to cool.
5. Add toasted pine nuts, feta cheese, cranberries, parsley, and lemon juice to the quinoa and broccoli. Mix everything together.

6. Serve the salad warm or chilled.
Prep Time: 30 minutes

Shrimp and Brown Rice Paella

Ingredients:
- 2 tablespoons of olive oil
- 1 onion, chopped
- 2 cloves of garlic, minced
- 1 red bell pepper, chopped
- 1 cup of long-grain brown rice
- 2 cups of chicken broth
- 1 teaspoon of smoked paprika
- 1/4 teaspoon of cayenne pepper
- 1/2 teaspoon of ground cumin
- 1/4 teaspoon of saffron threads
- 1 (14.5-ounce) can of diced tomatoes
- 1/2 pound of medium shrimp, peeled and deveined
- 1/4 cup of chopped fresh parsley
- 1 lemon, cut into wedges

Meal Preparation:
1. Heat the olive oil in a large skillet over medium heat. Add the onions and garlic, and cook until softened, about 5 minutes.
2. Add the bell pepper and cook for an additional 2 minutes.
3. Add the rice, stirring to coat with the oil. Cook for 2 minutes.
4. Pour in the chicken broth, smoked paprika, cayenne pepper, cumin, and saffron. Stir to combine, and bring to a simmer.
5. Reduce the heat to low, cover, and cook for 25 minutes.
6. Add the diced tomatoes and shrimp, stirring to combine. Cover and cook for an additional 10 minutes, or until the shrimp are cooked through.
7. Remove from the heat and stir in the parsley. Serve with lemon wedges.
Prep Time: 40 minutes
Turkey and White Bean Chili

Ingredients:
-1 pound ground turkey
-1 onion, diced
-1 bell pepper, diced
-3 cloves garlic, minced
-1 tablespoon chili powder
-1 teaspoon cumin
-1 teaspoon oregano
-1/2 teaspoon salt
-1/4 teaspoon black pepper
-1 (15 ounce) can white beans, drained and rinsed
-1 (14.5 ounce) can diced tomatoes
-1 cup chicken broth

Meal Preparation:
1. In a large pot, cook the ground turkey over medium-high heat until no longer pink.
2. Add the onion, bell pepper, and garlic. Cook until the vegetables are softened, about 5 minutes.
3. Add the chili powder, cumin, oregano, salt, and pepper. Stir to combine.
4. Add the white beans, tomatoes, and chicken broth. Stir to combine.
5. Bring the chili to a boil, then reduce the heat and simmer for 15 minutes, stirring occasionally.
Prep Time: 20 minutes

Baked Sweet Potato Fries

Ingredients:
2 sweet potatoes, cut into fries
2 tablespoons extra-virgin olive oil
1 teaspoon garlic powder
1/2 teaspoon paprika
1/4 teaspoon sea salt

Meal Preparation:

1. Preheat oven to 425°F and line a baking sheet with parchment paper.
2. In a large bowl, combine sweet potatoes, olive oil, garlic powder, paprika, and salt. Mix until evenly coated.
3. Spread fries on the baking sheet, making sure they are not overlapping.
4. Bake for 25-30 minutes, flipping once halfway through cooking time.
Prep Time: 10 minutes

Grilled Vegetable and Farro Salad

Ingredients:
-1/2 cup farro
-2 tablespoons olive oil
-1 red bell pepper, sliced
-1 zucchini, sliced
-1/2 cup cherry tomatoes, halved
-1/4 cup fresh parsley, chopped
-1/4 cup feta cheese, crumbled
-2 tablespoons red wine vinegar
-Salt and pepper to taste

Meal Preparation:
1. Preheat the grill to medium-high heat.
2. Rinse the farro and place in a medium saucepan. Cover with 2 cups of water and bring to a boil.
3. Reduce heat to low, cover and simmer for 15-20 minutes or until the farro is tender.
4. Drain the farro and place it in a large bowl.
5. Toss the bell pepper and zucchini slices with the olive oil and season with salt and pepper.
6. Grill the vegetables for 5-7 minutes, flipping once, or until lightly charred and tender.
7. Add the grilled vegetables, cherry tomatoes, parsley, feta cheese and red wine vinegar to the bowl with the farro.

8. Toss everything together and season with additional salt and pepper to taste.
Prep Time: 25 minutes

Turkey and Brown Rice Stuffed Peppers

Ingredients:
-1 cup cooked brown rice
-1 lb ground turkey
-1/3 cup chopped onion
-1 clove garlic, minced
-1 teaspoon dried oregano
-1/2 teaspoon dried basil
-1 teaspoon salt
-1/4 teaspoon ground black pepper
-1 (14.5 oz) can diced tomatoes, undrained
-4 large bell peppers
-1/2 cup shredded part-skim mozzarella cheese

Meal Preparation:
1. Preheat oven to 350°F
2. In a large skillet, cook the ground turkey, onion, garlic, oregano, basil, salt, and pepper over medium heat until the turkey is cooked through.
3. Add the cooked brown rice and diced tomatoes to the cooked turkey and stir until combined.
4. Cut the bell peppers in half and remove the tops, seeds, and membranes.
5. Place the peppers in a baking dish and fill with the turkey and rice mixture.
6. Top with the mozzarella cheese.
7. Bake in preheated oven for 35 minutes, or until the peppers are tender.
Prep Time: 20 minutes
Cook Time: 35 minutes

Roasted Cauliflower and Chickpea Curry

Ingredients:
• 1 head of cauliflower, cut into florets
• 2 cans of chickpeas, drained and rinsed
• 1 onion, diced
• 2 cloves of garlic, minced
• 1 teaspoon of ground cumin
• 1 teaspoon of ground coriander
• 1 teaspoon of garam masala
• 1 teaspoon of turmeric
• 1 can of coconut milk
• 2 tablespoons of olive oil
• Salt and pepper to taste

Meal Preparation:
1. Preheat the oven to 400 degrees Fahrenheit and line a baking sheet with parchment paper.
2. Place the cauliflower florets onto the baking sheet and drizzle with olive oil. Sprinkle with salt and pepper and toss to coat. Roast for 20 minutes, flipping once halfway through.
3. Meanwhile, heat a large skillet over medium-high heat and add the olive oil. Add the onion and garlic and sauté for 3-4 minutes until the onion is softened.
4. Add the chickpeas, cumin, coriander, garam masala, and turmeric to the skillet and stir to combine. Cook for another 3-4 minutes until the spices are fragrant.
5. Add the roasted cauliflower and coconut milk to the skillet and stir to combine. Reduce the heat to low and simmer for 10 minutes.
6. Taste and adjust seasoning as needed with salt and pepper. Serve over rice or quinoa.
Prep Time: 30 minutes

Grilled Salmon with Kale and Lemon

Ingredients:
- 2 salmon fillets

- 2 handfuls of kale, chopped
- 1 lemon, sliced
- 1 tablespoon olive oil
- Salt and pepper to taste

Meal Preparation:
1. Preheat the grill to medium heat.
2. Rub the salmon with the olive oil, salt, and pepper.
3. Place the salmon fillets on the grill and cook for 4-5 minutes per side, or until cooked through.
4. Place the chopped kale in a bowl and drizzle with olive oil.
5. Place the kale on the grill and cook for 3-4 minutes, or until lightly charred.
6. Place the salmon and kale on a plate and top with lemon slices.
Prep Time: 10 minutes

Stuffed Acorn Squash

Ingredients:
-2 acorn squash
-1 tablespoon olive oil
-1/2 cup cooked quinoa
-1/2 cup diced onion
-1/2 cup diced celery
-1/2 cup diced mushrooms
-1 cup cooked black beans
-1/2 cup crumbled feta cheese
-2 tablespoons chopped fresh parsley
-Salt and pepper to taste

Meal Preparation:
1. Preheat the oven to 400°F.
2. Cut squash in half and remove seeds. Brush squash with olive oil and season with salt and pepper.
3. Place squash cut-side down on a baking sheet and bake for 25 minutes.

4. Meanwhile, heat a large skillet over medium-high heat and add onion and celery. Saute until soft, about 5 minutes.
5. Add mushrooms and cook for an additional 2 minutes.
6. Add quinoa, black beans, feta cheese, parsley, salt and pepper and cook for an additional 3 minutes.
7. Remove squash from oven and fill each half with the quinoa mixture.
8. Return to oven and bake for an additional 15 minutes.
Prep Time: 45 minutes

Lentil and Spinach Soup

Ingredients:
-1 cup lentils
-1 onion, diced
-3 cloves garlic, minced
-2 carrots, diced
-2 stalks celery, diced
-1 teaspoon cumin
-1 teaspoon smoked paprika
-1/2 teaspoon dried oregano
-4 cups vegetable broth
-1 bunch spinach, chopped
-Salt and pepper, to taste

Meal Preparation:
1. In a medium saucepan, heat 1 tablespoon of olive oil over medium-high heat.
2. Add in the onion, garlic, carrots and celery. Cook for 5 minutes, stirring occasionally.
3. Add in the cumin, smoked paprika and oregano, stirring to combine.
4. Pour in the vegetable broth and lentils. Bring to a low boil, then reduce heat and simmer for 15-20 minutes, or until lentils are tender.
5. Add in the chopped spinach and cook for an additional 5 minutes.
6. Season with salt and pepper, to taste.
7. Serve hot.

Prep Time: 25 minutes

Quinoa and Black Bean Burger

Ingredients:
-1/2 cup uncooked quinoa
-1 can black beans, drained and rinsed
-1/2 cup diced onion
-1/2 cup diced bell pepper
-1/2 cup breadcrumbs
-1/4 cup chopped cilantro
-1/2 teaspoon cumin
-1/2 teaspoon chili powder
-1/4 teaspoon garlic powder
-1/4 teaspoon salt
-1/4 teaspoon pepper

Meal Preparation:
1. Preheat the oven to 350 degrees F.
2. Cook quinoa according to package instructions.
3. In a large bowl, mash black beans with a fork.
4. Add cooked quinoa, onion, bell pepper, breadcrumbs, cilantro, cumin, chili powder, garlic powder, salt, and pepper. Mix together until combined.
3. Form mixture into patties and place on a greased baking sheet.
4. Bake for 25 minutes, flipping halfway through.
Prep Time: 10 minutes
Cook Time: 25 minutes

Baked Apples with Walnuts and Cinnamon

Ingredients:
- 2 Apples
- 2 tablespoons Walnuts, chopped
- 2 teaspoons Cinnamon
- 2 tablespoons Maple Syrup

- 2 tablespoons Butter, melted
- 2 tablespoons Raisins (optional)

Meal Preparation:
1. Preheat the oven to 350°F (180°C).
2. Cut the apples in half and remove the cores. Place the apples in a baking dish.
3. In a small bowl, combine the walnuts, cinnamon, maple syrup, melted butter and raisins (if using).
4. Spoon the mixture into the center of each apple half.
5. Bake for 25-30 minutes, or until the apples are tender and the topping is golden brown.
Prep Time: 10 minutes
Cook Time: 25-30 minutes

Wild Rice and Mushroom Pilaf
Ingredients:
-1 cup wild rice
-1 cup long grain white rice
-2 tablespoons olive oil
-1 large onion, diced
-1 cup sliced mushrooms
-2 cloves garlic, minced
-2 cups vegetable broth
-1 teaspoon dried thyme
-Salt and pepper to taste

Meal Preparation:
1. Heat the olive oil in a large saucepan over medium heat.
2. Add the onion and mushrooms and cook for about 5 minutes, stirring occasionally, until the onion is softened.
3. Stir in the garlic and cook for 1 minute more.
4. Add the wild rice, white rice, vegetable broth, thyme, salt, and pepper.
5. Bring to a boil, then reduce heat to low and cover.

6. Simmer for 40 minutes, until the rice is tender and has absorbed all the liquid.
Prep Time: 15 minutes
Cook Time: 40 minutes

Butternut Squash Risotto

Ingredients:
-1 butternut squash, peeled and diced
-1 onion, diced
-3 cloves garlic, minced
-2 tablespoons olive oil
-1 cup arborio rice
-4 cups vegetable broth
-1/4 cup white wine
-1/4 cup grated Parmesan cheese
-2 tablespoons butter
-1 tablespoon chopped fresh sage
-Salt and pepper, to taste

Meal Preparation:
1. Heat the olive oil in a large pot over medium heat.
2. Add the onion and garlic and cook until softened, about 5 minutes.
3. Add the butternut squash and cook for an additional 3 minutes.
4. Add the arborio rice and stir to coat.
5. Add the vegetable broth and white wine, stirring to combine.
6. Bring the mixture to a boil, then reduce the heat to low and simmer for 15 minutes, stirring occasionally.
7. Add the Parmesan cheese, butter, and sage and stir to combine.
8. Season with salt and pepper, to taste.
9. Serve the risotto warm.
Prep Time: 25 minutes

Roasted Eggplant and Tomato Stacks
Ingredients:
-1 large eggplant, thinly sliced

-2 large tomatoes, thinly sliced
-1/2 cup grated Parmesan cheese
-Olive oil
-Salt and pepper

Meal Preparation:
1. Preheat the oven to 375 degrees F.
2. Arrange the eggplant slices on a large baking sheet and brush with olive oil.
3. Sprinkle with salt and pepper.
4. Place the tomato slices on top of the eggplant slices, and brush with olive oil.
5. Sprinkle with Parmesan cheese.
6. Bake for 20 minutes, or until the eggplant is tender and the cheese is golden brown.
Prep Time: 10 minutes
Cook Time: 20 minutes

Turkey and Vegetable Meatloaf

Ingredients:

-1 lb ground turkey
-1/2 cup diced onion
-1/2 cup diced red bell pepper
-1/2 cup diced celery
-1/2 cup Italian-style bread crumbs
-1/4 cup ketchup
-1 egg
-1 tsp garlic powder
-1/2 tsp salt
-1/4 tsp black pepper

Meal Preparation:
1. Preheat oven to 350°F.

2. In a large bowl, combine ground turkey, onion, bell pepper,
celery, bread crumbs, ketchup, egg, garlic powder, salt, and pepper.
3. Mix all ingredients together until fully combined.
4. Form mixture into a loaf shape and transfer it to a lightly greased
9x5-inch loaf pan.
5. Bake in preheated oven for 45 minutes, or until the internal
temperature of the meatloaf has reached 165°F.
Prep Time: 15 minutes
Cook Time: 45 minutes

Roasted Asparagus and Red Pepper Quiche

Ingredients:
- 1/2 bunch of asparagus, trimmed
- 1 red bell pepper, cut into thin strips
- 1/2 cup chopped onion
- 1/2 cup shredded cheese
- 5 eggs
- 1/2 cup milk
- 1/4 teaspoon salt
- 1/4 teaspoon pepper
- 1/2 teaspoon dried oregano
- 1/2 teaspoon garlic powder

Meal Preparation:
1. Preheat the oven to 375 degrees F.
2. Grease a 9-inch pie dish with butter or cooking spray.
3. Arrange the asparagus and bell pepper strips in the bottom of the
pie dish.
4. Sprinkle the chopped onion, cheese, and spices over the
vegetables.
5. In a separate bowl, whisk together the eggs, milk, salt, and pepper
until combined.
6. Pour the egg mixture over the vegetables in the pie dish.
7. Bake for 40-45 minutes, or until the quiche is golden brown and a
knife inserted into the center comes out clean.

Prep time: 10 minutes
Cook time: 40-45 minutes

JUICE RECIPES

1. Beet, Carrot and Apple Juice
2. Kale, Spinach and Celery Juice
3. Carrot, Ginger and Orange Juice
4. Beet, Apple and Pear Juice
5. Apple and Celery Juice
6. Apple, Cucumber and Lemon Juice
7. Carrot, Parsley and Orange Juice
8. Pineapple, Cucumber and Mint Juice
9. Carrot, Spinach and Apple Juice
10. Beet, Cucumber and Apple Juice
11. Orange and Grapefruit Juice
12. Apple, Cucumber and Kale Juice
13. Carrot, Orange and Ginger Juice
14. Spinach and Apple Juice
15. Blueberry, Banana and Almond Milk Juice
16. Pear and Mint Juice
17. Beet, Carrot and Orange Juice
18. Apple, Celery and Parsley Juice
19. Carrot, Lemon and Ginger Juice

Beet, Carrot and Apple Juice

Ingredients:
-3 beets
-2 carrots
-2 apples

Meal Preparation:
1. Wash and peel the beets, carrots, and apples.
2. Cut the beets, carrots, and apples into small pieces.
3. Place the pieces into a blender and blend until smooth.
4. Strain the juice through a fine mesh strainer.
5. Pour the juice into a glass and enjoy!
Prep Time: 15 minutes

Kale, Spinach and Celery Juice

Ingredients:
- 2 beets
- 2 carrots
- 2 apples

Meal Preparation:
1. Wash and peel the beets, carrots, and apples.
2. Cut the beets, carrots, and apples into small pieces.
3. Place the pieces into a juicer and blend until smooth.
Prep Time:15 minutes

Carrot, Ginger and Orange Juice

Ingredients:
- 2 carrots, peeled and cubed
- 1 inch piece of fresh ginger, peeled and minced
- 1 orange, juiced

Meal Preparation:
1. Place the cubed carrots in a blender and blend until smooth.

2. Add the minced ginger to the carrots and blend until fully combined.
3. Squeeze the juice from the orange into the carrot-ginger mixture and blend until fully incorporated.
Prep Time: 10 minutes

Beet, Apple and Pear Juice

Ingredients:
- 2 beets
- 2 apples
- 2 pears

Meal Preparation:
1. Wash and peel the beets, apples, and pears.
2. Chop the beets, apples, and pears into small pieces.
3. Place the chopped pieces into a juicer and process until all the juice is extracted.
4. Strain the juice through a fine-mesh strainer to remove any pulp.
5. Serve the juice chilled.
Prep Time: 15 minutes

Apple and Celery Juice

Ingredients:
-1 apple
-2 stalks of celery

Meal Preparation:
1. Wash the apple and celery stalks.
2. Cut the apple into slices and the celery into thin strips.
3. Put both the apple slices and celery strips into a blender.
4. Add a cup of water and blend until smooth.
5. Strain the juice into a glass and serve.
Prep Time: 10 minutes

Apple, Cucumber and Lemon Juice

Ingredients:

- 2 apples
- 1 cucumber
- 1 lemon

Meal Preparation:
1. Wash the apples and cucumber with cold water.
2. Peel the apples and cucumber.
3. Cut the apples, cucumber and lemon into small pieces.
4. Put the pieces into a blender and blend until smooth.
5. Pour the mixture through a strainer to remove any remaining pulp.
6. Place the strained juice into a glass and enjoy.
Prep Time: 15 minutes
Carrot, Parsley and Orange Juice
Ingredients:
-Carrots (2-3)
-Parsley (1 handful)
-Orange Juice (1 cup)

Meal Preparation:
1. Wash and peel the carrots.
2. Chop the carrots into small cubes.
3. Wash and chop the parsley.
4. Put the carrots, parsley and orange juice into a blender.
5. Blend until smooth.
Prep Time: 10 minutes

Pineapple, Cucumber and Mint Juice

Ingredients:
- 2 cups fresh pineapple chunks
- 2 cucumbers, peeled and chopped

- 1/4 cup fresh mint leaves
Meal Preparation:

1. Place the pineapple chunks, cucumbers and mint leaves in a blender.
2. Blend until all ingredients are well combined, about 1 minute.
3. Strain the juice through a fine mesh sieve, pressing down on the solids to extract as much juice as possible.
Prep Time: 10 minutes

Carrot, Spinach and Apple Juice

Ingredients:
- 2 carrots
- 2 apples
- 2 handfuls of spinach

Meal Preparation:
1. Wash and peel the carrots and apples.
2. Cut them into small pieces.
3. Put the carrots, apples and spinach into a blender.
4. Blend until smooth.
5. Strain the juice through a fine mesh sieve and discard the solid pieces.
Prep Time: 10 minutes

Beet, Cucumber and Apple Juice

Ingredients:
-1 beet, peeled and chopped
-1 cucumber, peeled and chopped
-1 apple, cored and chopped

Meal Preparation:
-Wash the beet, cucumber, and apple with cold water.

-Peel and chop the beet, cucumber, and apple into small pieces.
-Place the chopped beet, cucumber, and apple into a juicer and process until smooth.
Prep Time: 10 minutes

Apple, Cucumber and Kale Juice

Ingredients:
- 1 apple
- ½ cucumber
- 1 cup of kale

Meal Preparation:
1. Wash and cut the apple into small pieces.
2. Peel and cut the cucumber into small pieces.
3. Wash the kale and remove any tough stems.
4. Place the apple, cucumber, and kale pieces into a blender.
5. Blend until smooth.
6. Strain the juice into a glass.
Prep Time: 10 minutes

Orange and Grapefruit Juice

Ingredients:
• 2 oranges
• 2 grapefruits

Meal Preparation:

1. Wash and peel the oranges and grapefruits.
2. Cut the fruits into small pieces.
3. Put the pieces into a blender and blend until it becomes a juice.
4. Strain the juice through a sieve to remove any pulp or seeds.
Prep Time:10 minutes

Carrot, Orange and Ginger Juice

Ingredients:
- 2 large carrots, peeled and roughly chopped
- 1 large orange, peeled and roughly chopped
- 1 inch piece of fresh ginger, peeled and roughly chopped

Meal Preparation:

1. Place all ingredients into a blender and blend until smooth.
2. Strain the mixture through a sieve and discard the solids.
3. Pour the juice into a glass and enjoy.
Prep Time: 10 minutes

Spinach and Apple Juice

Ingredients
- 1 cup spinach
- 2 apples

Meal Preparation
1. Wash the spinach and apples in cold water.
2. Peel and core the apples.
3. Chop the spinach and apples into small pieces.
4. Place the chopped pieces into a blender.
5. Blend until combined into a smooth juice.
Prep Time: 10 minutes

Blueberry, Banana and Almond Milk Juice

Ingredients:
-1 cup blueberries
-1 banana
-1 cup almond milk

Meal Preparation:
-Wash the blueberries and banana.
-Peel the banana.
-Place the blueberries and bananas into a blender.
-Pour in the almond milk.
-Blend the ingredients until smooth.
Prep Time: 5 minutes

Pear and Mint Juice

Ingredients:
-2 pears, peeled, cored and cut into pieces
-1/2 cup of fresh mint leaves
-1 cup of cold water
-2 tablespoons of honey

Meal Preparation:
1. Place the pear pieces in a blender and blend until smooth.
2. Add the mint leaves, cold water, and honey and blend until all ingredients are combined.
3. Strain the juice into a pitcher.
4. Serve the juice chilled or over ice.
Prep Time: 10 minutes

Beet, Carrot and Orange Juice

Ingredients:
- 2 beets
- 2 carrots
- 2 oranges

Meal Preparation:
1. Wash the beets, carrots, and oranges under cool running water.
2. Peel the beets and carrots using a vegetable peeler.
3. Cut the beets and carrots into pieces that fit in the juicer.
4. Cut the oranges in half and remove the seeds.

5. Put the beets, carrots, and oranges into the juicer and juice them until all the juice has been extracted.
6. Pour the juice into a glass and enjoy.
Prep Time: 10 minutes

Apple, Celery and Parsley Juice

Ingredients:
- 2 apples
- 2 stalks of celery
- 1 handful of parsley

Meal Preparation:
1. Wash and core the apples, celery and parsley.
2. Cut the apples and celery into small pieces.
3. Place the apples, celery and parsley into a blender.
4. Blend on high speed until the mixture is smooth.
5. Serve in a glass.
Prep Time: 10 minutes
Carrot, Lemon and Ginger Juice

Ingredients:
-3 large carrots
-1 large lemon
-2-inch piece of fresh ginger

Meal Preparation:
-Wash and peel carrots, lemon, and ginger
-Cut carrots, lemon and ginger into small pieces
-Put all the pieces into a blender and blend until smooth
Prep Time: 10 minutes

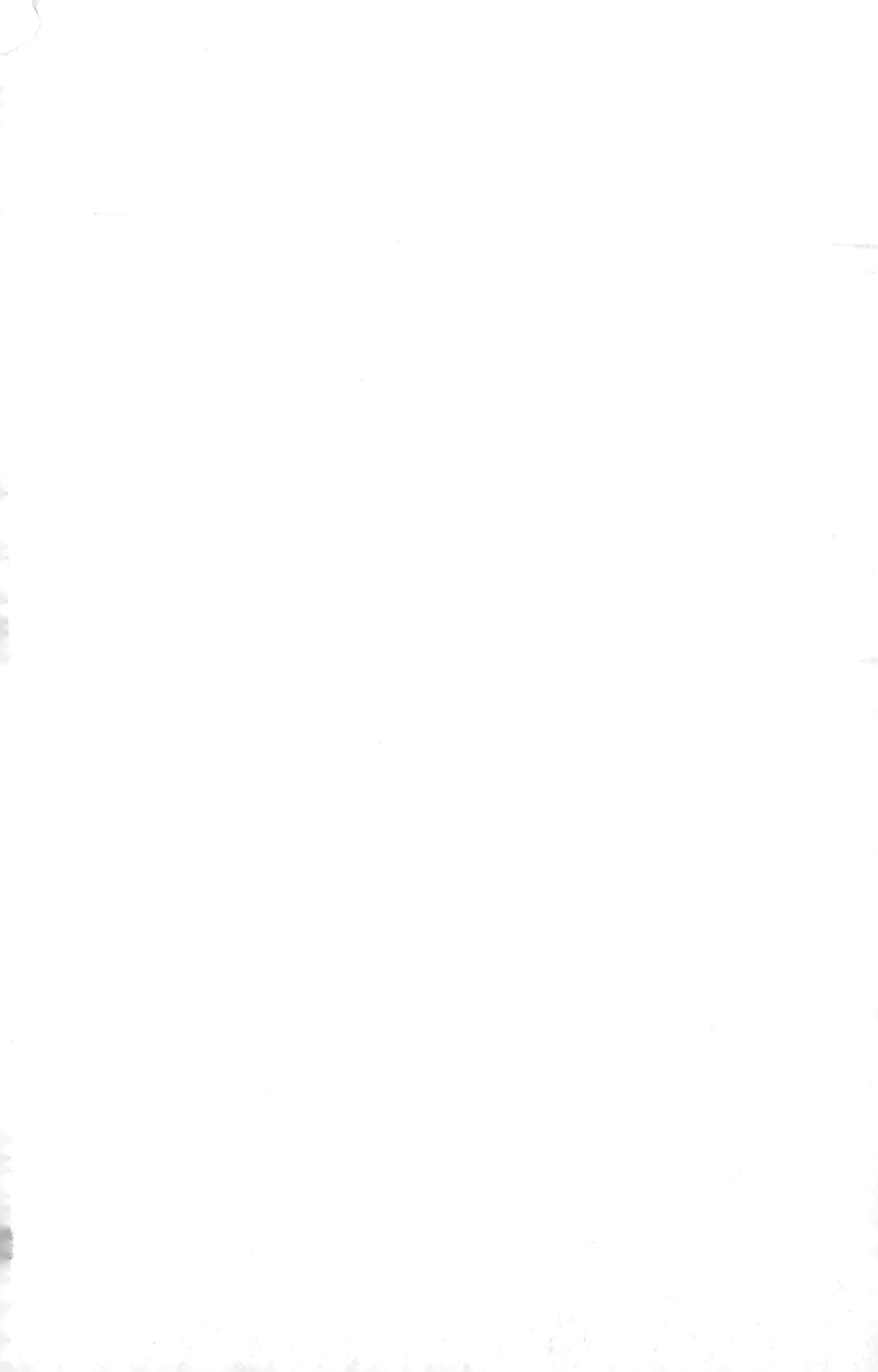